Handbook of
CLINICAL TRIALS

Marcus Flather

Hazel Aston

Rod Stables

ReMEDICAPUBLISHING

CONTRIBUTORS

Steve Aldis BSc, MSc
Formerly IT Professional, CTEU

Hazel Aston MSc
Clinical Research Co-ordinator, CTEU

Ameet Bakhai MRCP
Senior Clinical Research Fellow, CTEU
Specialist Registrar in Cardiology, Royal Brompton and
Harefield NHS Trust; Honorary Lecturer, Imperial College
of Science, Technology and Medicine, London, UK

Ian Barnes BSc
Formerly Clinical Research Co-ordinator, CTEU

Jean Booth BSc, MSc, RGN
Senior Clinical Scientist, CTEU

Pauline Dooley
Formerly Head of Unit Administration, CTEU

Marcus Flather BSc, MBBS, FRCP
Director, CTEU; Honorary Consultant, Royal Brompton
and Harefield NHS Trust; Senior Lecturer, Imperial College
of Science, Technology and Medicine, London, UK

Belinda Lees BSc, PhD
Senior Clinical Research Co-ordinator, CTEU and
Imperial College of Science, Technology and Medicine

Rebecca Mister BSc
Clinical Research Co-ordinator, CTEU

Handbook of
CLINICAL
TRIALS

ReMEDICAPUBLISHING

Published by ReMEDICA Publishing Limited
32-38 Osnaburgh Street, London, NW1 3ND, UK

Tel: +44 20 7388 7677
Fax: +44 20 7388 7457
Email: books@remedica.com
www.remedica.com

ISBN 1 901346 29 3

British Library Cataloguing-in-Publication Data
A catalogue record for this book is available from the British Library.

Fiona Nugara BSc
Data Manager, CTEU

Diego Perez de Arenaza MBBS
Research Fellow, CTEU and Hospital Italiano
de Buenos Aires, Buenos Aires, Argentina

Marcelo Shibata MD
Senior Research Fellow, CTEU and Institute of Health
Economics, Edmonton, Canada; Consultant Cardiologist,
Instituto Dante Pazzanese de Cardiologia, Sao Paulo, Brazil

Rod Stables MA, MRCP
Formerly Deputy Director, CTEU, now Consultant
Cardiologist, The Cardiothoracic Centre,
Thomas Drive, Liverpool L14 3PE, UK

Marrianne Stuteville BSc
Formerly Clinical Research Co-ordinator, CTEU,
now Clinical Co-ordinator Stents, Guidant Europe

Duolao Wang PhD
Lecturer, Medical Statistics Unit, London School
of Hygiene and Tropical Medicine, Keppel Street,
London WC1E 7HT, UK

We acknowledge the support of Matthew Forster,
Lynette Batt, Nicola Delahunty and Tugayel Khan of CTEU.

Please address all correspondence to:
c/o Dr Marcus Flather, Royal Brompton Hospital,
Clinical Trials and Evaluation Unit,
Sydney Street, London, SW3 6NP, UK

CONTENTS

PREFACE

PROFESSOR ANTHONY NEWMAN TAYLOR

Well-designed randomized trials have become an essential basis for evidence-informed clinical practice: most modern therapeutic advances have come from the results of such trials, which have appropriately been described as the 'gold standard' for clinical evidence.

This handbook provides essential information for anyone wanting to participate in a multicenter clinical trial. Chapters on trial design and statistics provide important theory; more practical information is provided in the chapters on the regulatory process, participating in trials and data management. It is now 50 years since the early landmark trials of Bradford Hill, but much of the methodology, logic and statistical assumptions remain valid. We must never lose sight of the research question: a well-conducted trial will only be as important as the clinical question it addresses. This handbook will stimulate health professionals to think more about the rationale for trials and the best way for these to be conducted to the highest standards. The expertise of the Clinical Trials and Evaluation Unit has produced an excellent handbook that will become valuable reading for any involved in clinical trials.

Professor Newman Taylor OBE is Director of Research at the Royal Brompton and Harefield NHS Trust and Professor of Occupational and Environmental Medicine at the National Heart and Lung Institute of Imperial College of Science, Technology and Medicine.

INTRODUCTION

HAZEL ASTON, MARCUS FLATHER, ROD STABLES

This book covers the important aspects of participating in multicenter clinical trials and is aimed at health professionals with an interest in clinical research. New investigators and those with some experience will benefit from the comprehensive range of topics covered in the book. It is not intended as a comprehensive textbook but rather as a handbook of practical issues. The chapters of the book can be read consecutively or consulted individually as an easy reference as the need arises. The content material covers all the major aspects of setting up and running trials including trial design, statistics, financial issues, ethics and regulatory requirements. In each chapter key points are highlighted in tables and diagrams. This design allows rapid assimilation of important information particularly when using the book as reference.

Many aspects of multicenter clinical trials, including regulatory and ethical issues, are changing rapidly. Appropriate web site references are provided for these issues, and the reader is encouraged to review these for the latest information. We hope that readers will let us know about errors and omissions.

The book has been the result of a collaboration of personnel in the Clinical Trials and Evaluation Unit of the Royal Brompton and Harefield NHS Trust, London, UK. The Editors would like to thank all contributors for their diligence, hard work and patience in producing the final version of the book. We would also like to thank our publisher ReMEDICA, especially Andrew Ward and Tamsin White for their support and advice during the production of the book.

CHAPTER 1

Design issues in observational studies and randomized trials

Marcelo Shibata, Marcus Flather & Diego Perez de Arenaza

Introduction

A variety of study designs are used in clinical research. Different designs are appropriate in different circumstances, and each can provide useful data. It is important for the study investigator to understand the advantages and disadvantages of each type of study to enable him/her to apply them appropriately and to interpret the results.

Study designs in clinical research

Observational
- Case report
- Case series
- Cross-sectional survey
- Case control
- Cohort studies

Randomized
- Clinical trials

Observational study designs

Observational methods for data collection (outcome studies, performance tables and audit) are useful descriptive tools, but cannot reliably compare the effects of different treatments because of inherent biases. These biases arise from an inability to control for numerous confounding factors between comparison groups.

In general, observational studies generate hypotheses for further investigation, rather than answering questions about treatment effects. For example well-designed cohort studies may give powerful insights into disease etiology. Allocating treatments using randomization generally allows unbiased statistical comparisons to be made between groups that are matched for known and unknown prognostic factors.

Case reports and case series

A case report describes interesting or relevant aspects of a single case, such as an unusual episode of poisoning or an atypical rash developing after the administration of a new medication. Case reports detailing the occurrence of Kaposi's sarcoma (a malignant, vascular proliferative condition normally found in older men) in a group of young homosexual men who had a history of sexually transmitted diseases, were the first recognition of AIDS as a new clinical syndrome[1]. Thus, these observational methods can be useful for sharing experiences with other colleagues and identifying potentially important avenues for further investigation.

Case series are groups of case reports comprising similar observations, or using similar treatments or procedures, usually in consecutive patients. A case series may be an important way to establish a new surgical method (see Chapter 2), especially if there is a pre-specified protocol for the study. Unfortunately, most case series are retrospective in nature (i.e. the idea for the case series occurs after most, or all, of the procedures have been carried out), and these studies usually suffer from incomplete data collection and analysis.

Key Points: Case Reports and Case Series

Definition: a case report is a brief description of a single case that an observer feels should be brought to the attention of colleagues. Case series are several case reports of similar observations or procedures that can be grouped together.

Advantages
- Simple to perform
- Reports may be written up and published rapidly

Disadvantages
- Limited insights about disease etiology or treatment efficacy
- Difficult to make reliable comparisons of treatment effects
- Retrospective case series may contain incomplete data

Cross-sectional surveys

The cross-sectional approach begins with selection of a particular population or cohort. Patient characteristics, treatments and prevalence of disease are then documented within the cohort. These observations are used to identify any associations between potential risk factors and the disease of interest **(Figure 1)**.

Cross-sectional surveys are performed at a single point in time. If patients are followed for any period of time, then the study becomes a cohort study (see below). Surveys may be conducted using sampling methods that allow results to be generalized to larger populations.

Surveys are useful for gaining information about the characteristics of patients with a particular syndrome and how to manage patients. They may also be used to generate hypotheses for further investigation.

Clinical audit is a type of cross-sectional survey. Audit is a term given to collection of information about patients, treatments and outcomes in routine clinical practice. Unfortunately, audit has been a difficult exercise to carry out in many clinical areas due to a lack of the resources and staff required to maintain data collection and analysis.

Key Points: Cross-Sectional Survey

Definition: a cross-sectional survey is a study in which simultaneous assessments of outcomes, descriptive features and potential predictors are made.

Advantages
- Inexpensive and simple to carry out
- No follow-up required
- Possible to estimate the frequency of a disease within a group

Disadvantages
- Does not provide information about longer term outcomes

Case control studies

Case control studies utilize retrospective comparisons to generate hypotheses about disease etiology. Patients who already have a particular disease are compared with individuals who do not have the disease (**Figure 2**). For example, a case control study may be carried out by studying patients who developed eclampsia during their pregnancy (case) and patients who did not (control). A search for risk factors related to the occurrence of eclampsia is then performed, and a comparison of potential etiological factors is made between the cases and controls. However, the choice of an appropriate control group often

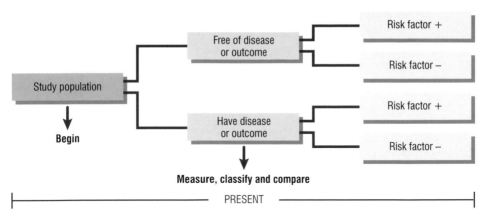

FIGURE 1. Cross-sectional survey

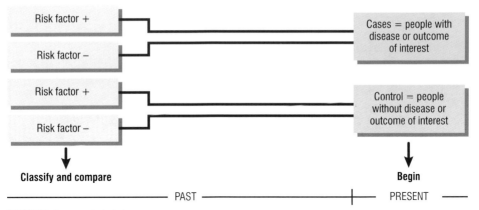

FIGURE 2. Case control study

proves difficult. The control group should be selected from individuals who have been 'exposed' to the same environment as the case group. Otherwise, there is potential for bias in the study results by selectively including subjects who either underestimate or overestimate exposures.

In general, controls are 'matched' to the case group for age, gender and ethnic origin. Other factors such as residential location, weight, height and so on, can also be matched. There are no clear guidelines on the extent of matching required in a case control study.

Key Points: Case Control Studies

Definition: case control studies begin by identifying individuals with a particular disease or outcome (case) and those without it (control). Comparisons of possible etiological factors in the subjects' histories are then carried out.

Advantages
- Simple to perform
- Can generate useful hypotheses of disease etiology
- Feasible method to study rare diseases, or situations in which there is a long lag between exposure and outcome

Disadvantages
- Retrospective research
- Usually relies on searching health records that may be incomplete or biased
- Not all risk factors related to disease or outcome may be taken into account
- Identification of controls and degree of matching may be problematic

Prospective cohort studies

Prospective cohort studies begin with the selection of a group of individuals who do not have the disease or outcome of interest. The individuals are then examined and classified using certain characteristics, which might be related to the outcome. This prospectively defined cohort is then followed to determine who develops the disease or outcome of interest **(Figure 3)**.

A good example of a cohort study design is the British Doctors Study[2] set up in 1951 to assess possible etiological factors for lung cancer in 34,439 participants. This was the first large study to establish a strong association between smoking and lung cancer. The cohort has been followed up for 40 years through regular questionnaires. Approximately 10,000 subjects died during the first 20 years (1951–1971) and another 10,000 died during the second half of the study (1971–1991). The death-rate ratio of smokers to non-smokers during 1971–1991 was approximately three-fold at ages 45–64 and two-fold at ages 65–84.

Key Points: Cohort Study

Definition: a cohort study identifies a group (cohort) of people who have not experienced the disease or outcome of interest. The subjects are then followed to compare the incidence of disease between groups who have, or do not have, particular risk factors.

Advantages
- Subjects can be matched for possible confounding variables
- Eligibility criteria and outcomes can be standardized
- Insights about etiology can be made

Disadvantages
- Disease or outcome may be related to unidentified risk factors
- Follow-up may take many years for sufficient numbers of patients to manifest the disease of interest
- Most associations are merely hypothesis generating unless very strong

---

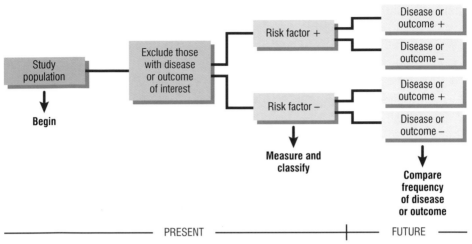

FIGURE 3. Cohort study

Randomized controlled trials

An important feature that distinguishes randomized trials from observational studies is the evaluation of a therapeutic intervention. Randomized trials are also known as interventional trials, but this term is now more commonly used for trials that evaluate invasive or surgical procedures. Randomization is a process used for allocating treatments to two or more groups of subjects, i.e. each subject is allocated his/her treatment by chance. This allows the treatment groups to be balanced for known and unknown variables that may influence the disease process and response to treatment. This supposition of 'balanced' groups is fundamental to the statistical assumptions made when analyzing randomized trials.

Most trials use pre-prepared treatment allocation lists generated from random number tables. To reduce the chance of selection bias in the allocation of treatments it is important that investigators in the trial do not know the identity of the next treatment allocation. This is called concealed or 'true' randomization.

In a randomized trial, eligible patients are randomly allocated to an active treatment group or a control group. The efficacy of treatment is measured after a pre-defined follow-up period **(Figure 4)**. Well-designed and conducted trials are the most reliable way to evaluate the safety and efficacy of new treatments.

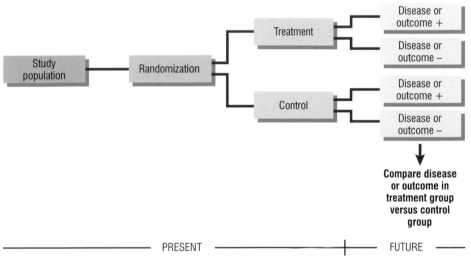

FIGURE 4. Randomized controlled trial

Clinical trials evaluate the effects of treatments in a controlled situation, therefore the enrolled patients may not be representative of a broader population with the same condition in clinical practice.

For these reasons a wide range of information beyond the clinical trial data is helpful when implementing new therapies. This includes the size and characteristics of the population to be treated, costs and other health economic issues, and an assessment of the practical aspects of using the new treatment in clinical practice.

Key protocol issues in randomized trials

Blinding

Blinding is a technique used to avoid bias during data collection and assessment. Several aspects of a trial can be blinded, such as the identity of the intervention, and the assessment, classification and evaluation of the response variables. There are three common types of 'blinded' clinical trials:

1. Unblinded ('open')

Both the investigator and the subject know which treatment has been assigned. There are some trials that can only be carried out in this manner, such as trials of surgical procedures (see chapter 2), learning techniques or changes in life style. Unblinded studies are simple in design but involve the possibility of bias, e.g. a subject in the treatment group may be more likely to report side effects than a subject in the control group.

2. Single-blind

Only the investigator is aware of which intervention each subject is receiving. Investigator bias in the conduct, analysis and reporting of the trial is a potential problem.

3. Double-blind (sometimes referred to as the 'double-dummy' technique)

Neither the investigator nor the subject knows the identity of the administered intervention. These studies use dummy (placebo) treatment for the control group. Double-blind study designs are more commonly used in trials of drug efficacy. The main advantage of this design is the reduction of bias as treatment effects and outcomes are reported without knowledge of the treatment allocation.

Key Points: Blinding of Study Treatments

- Ideally, both investigator and subject should be blinded to treatment allocation so as to avoid bias during data collection and assessment
- Blinding can be applied to several steps in a trial

Categories of blinding:

- Unblinded studies: both investigator and subject know to which intervention the latter has been assigned
- Single-blind studies: only the investigator is aware of which intervention each subject is receiving
- Double-blind studies: identity of treatment allocation is hidden from both the investigator and the subject

Eligibility

Eligibility defines the types of patients studied in a clinical trial. Eligibility criteria should be simple and unambiguous, thus facilitating recruitment and appropriately reflecting the conditions of patients seen in day-to-day practice. Broad eligibility criteria help to ensure that results can be generalized to clinical practice.

The inclusion criteria, and reasons for their use, should be stated in advance. Exclusion criteria should apply to subjects with a low probability of benefit, or those who may have a higher risk of adverse outcomes if entered into the trial. Extensive exclusion criteria (e.g. >10) often make it difficult to find patients to enroll in the trial.

> **Key Points: Eligibility**
> - Eligibility defines the subject's characteristics or disease of interest to be studied
> - Eligibility criteria should be simple and precisely specified without too many exclusions

Outcome measures

The trial protocol should clearly define the desired outcomes and how they are to be measured. Binary outcomes (an outcome measure that can assume only one of two values) such as mortality are robust, but require large studies to detect differences between treatment allocations. Most binary outcomes require special definitions for trial purposes, e.g. the definition of myocardial infarction is currently under review. Some research groups have proposed definitions based on biochemical markers, while others want to retain some elements of the clinical diagnosis.

Measurement of 'continuous' data, such as blood pressure, blood cholesterol or left ventricular function, require carefully designed protocols for the experimental methods. For example, assessment of the efficacy of an anti-hypertensive drug requires that the measurement of blood pressure be standardized in all study centers, including patient position, resting time before any measurement, number of readings at each patient visit, time from the last dose and calibration of the equipment.

> **Key Points: Outcome measures**
> - The trial protocol should clearly define the outcome events and how they will be measured
> - Outcome measures should be objective and simple to ascertain, in order to enhance the reliability of the results

Summary

We have outlined important design issues in observational and randomized trials. Well-designed prospective research, using appropriate methodology, can give valuable insights into disease etiology and treatment effects. All research projects should give adequate care and attention to design issues as these have a major impact on the quality and validity of the results.

References

1. Hymes KB, Greene JB, Marcus A et al. Kaposi's sarcoma in homosexual men-a report of eight cases. Lancet 1981;**2**:598.
2. Doll R, Peto R, Wheatley K et al. Mortality in relation to smoking: 40 years' observations on male British doctors. Br Med J 1994;**309**:901–11.

Suggested further reading

Pocock SJ. Clinical Trials: A Practical Approach. Wiley and Sons Ltd. 1983.
Ferguson FR, Davey AFC, Topley WWC. The value of mixed vaccines in the prevention of common cold. J Hyg 1927;**26**:98–109
Friedman LM, Furberg CD, DeMets DL. Fundamentals of Clinical Trials. Mosby-Year Book, Inc. 1985.
Sacket DL, Haynes BR, Guyatt GH et al. Clinical Epidemiology, a Basic Science for Clinical Medicine. Little Brown and Company. 1991.
Gehlbach SH. Interpreting the Medical Literature. McGraw-Hill, Inc. 1993.

CHAPTER 2

Design issues in the evaluation of surgical or interventional procedures

Rod Stables

Introduction

Regulatory authorities responsible for approval of a new drug or device demand high-quality evidence of efficacy and safety as part of the licensing process. More recently, health care purchasers (and individual patients) have begun to demand evidence to support the allocation of scarce resources to specific treatment strategies.

Although the concept and methodology of 'evidence-based practice' was framed in the context of drug therapy, the same principles apply in the evaluation of surgical or interventional procedures. Advances in technology and manufacturing have led to rapid development of new equipment and techniques, e.g. in the field of vascular intervention, the volume of new product registration in the USA is second only to that from the field of information technology. The need to test these new products, to refine their application and to define suitable patient populations has led to a near exponential growth in interventional research activity and 'procedure trials'.

Unfortunately, the randomized controlled trial (RCT) methodology, so elegant in the assessment of drug therapy, does not readily translate to the evaluation of surgical or interventional procedures, and a number of issues demand special consideration.

Evolution, refinement and dissemination of a new procedure

A new procedure or operation tends to follow a typical evolution over many years **(Figure 1)**. Initial experimental or animal work precedes the first human applications. Thereafter, the development of the first case series is often restricted to a single center, usually in the hands of a single operator. Commercial organizations are increasingly engaging a small number of centers in the initial evaluation of a new device or procedure. Even with this approach, the body of evidence accumulated at this stage remains scant.

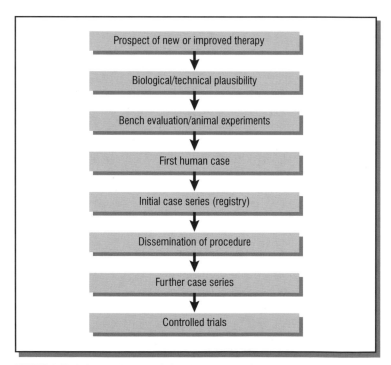

FIGURE 1. Typical stages in the evolution of a new procedure

As the technique becomes more widely disseminated, more procedures are performed and more operators become familiar with the technique.

The 'learning curve' effect

It is an established fact that the clinical results of a new procedure are less favorable in the initial stages of its development than when it is applied as a mature therapy. This 'learning curve' effect is multi-factorial in causation. Accumulated experience allows continuous refinement of patient selection, operative technique, adjunctive medication and post-procedural care. There are also operator and institutional aspects to this phenomenon as, even after the most fastidious period of training and preparation, performance tends to improve with additional practice.

The timing of evaluation

The inevitable consequence of this protracted period of development is that if a new procedure is subjected to formal evaluation too early in its 'natural history', then adverse clinical results may condemn a technique with great potential. If, however, the procedure is allowed to become too well established, then it may have gained such acceptance with doctors and patients that it becomes difficult to mount an RCT to compare it to previous generation therapy or to a conservative approach.

The value of case series (registry) evaluations

Although RCT methodology remains the best method for the assessment of a new therapy, the case series (or registry) is of considerable value in the development of a new procedure or operation. This approach allows a practical, rapid and cost-effective assessment of a developing strategy. Also, there is the potential for scientific rigor with the use of unselected, consecutive patients and the prospective definition of outcome measures. Results can be compared with historical controls or results from other centers, although this involves the potential for observed or unrecognized bias. Perhaps their greatest value is that they help to frame questions for future RCTs and the clinical conditions under which they will be addressed.

An individual or institutional case series provides a continuous record that grows over time. This is a useful source for subsequent retrospective research and allows operators to make a more precise statement of expected outcomes and risks for an individual patient, manifesting a certain pattern of clinical characteristics.

A case series can:
- help to frame questions for future RCTs
- form a useful source for retrospective research

RCTs for operations or procedures

In procedural RCTs the absence of a traditional 'drug type' placebo presents special problems. Most studies involve either:

- the head to head assessment of two different procedures, or
- a comparison of the experimental procedure against conventional (often conservative) therapy

It is usually impossible to blind either the patient or the clinical team to the treatment received. This presents problems in the assessment of outcome measures, which may be influenced by the 'open design'. For example, consider the recent trials of percutaneous myocardial revascularization by laser. Patients with chronic, intractable angina were randomized to the new procedure or continued medical therapy. The patient's reported symptoms at

Problems with RCTs for operations or procedures:

difficulties in 'blinding' the patient/operator

it is difficult to provide an appropriate 'placebo' for dramatic surgical/interventional procedures, thus any controls are generally 'non-treatment' groups

care may differ between treatment groups when evaluating different therapies

markedly different therapies requiring specialized techniques may be carried out by different operators thus differences in care may be observed

low recruitment rates

patient and operator preferences may affect recruitment rates

follow-up could be influenced by the attitude to having received the dramatic intervention or having simply continued as before.

Evaluation of markedly different therapies

The application of markedly different therapies can have other effects unrelated to the actual nature of the interventions, e.g. pre- and post-procedural care may differ between the two treatment groups. In trials comparing percutaneous transluminal coronary angioplasty (PTCA) and coronary artery bypass grafting (CABG) it has been suggested that care by cardiologists rather than cardiac surgeons may be associated with better application of secondary prevention measures. This might then influence the medium-term outcome, independent of the initial revascularization procedure allocated at randomization.

Pragmatic trial design

Advantages

- reflects clinical reality
- accommodates evolution in therapy
- trial procedures simplified
- minimal protocol restriction

Disadvantages

- multiple variations in details of therapy
- diverse patient population
- conclusions cannot be generalized

Trials offering randomization between two very different therapies (for example CABG and PTCA) are also vulnerable to low recruitment rates. Patient and operator preferences may result in few patients being approached and, even if attempted, the process of informed consent can be difficult. A low ratio of eligible patients screened to those randomized threatens the external validity of trial findings and limits the ability to generalize results to routine practice. In addition, the fact that intervention trials are generally carried out in a relatively small number of specialized centers with restrictive patient selection criteria further exacerbates this problem. In the early PTCA versus CABG trials as few as 2–5% of patients screened were entered in the studies.

Coping with changing treatment patterns

When a procedure is in a state of continuous evolution, trials can be initiated using techniques, devices or adjunctive medication schedules that are subsequently rendered obsolete. The concepts of 'moving goal posts' and studies 'overtaken by events' can hinder recruitment to ongoing studies and render the results of completed studies less relevant to current practice.

One approach to this problem is the concept of pragmatic trial design. This type of study aims to test a broad strategy approach and has very few protocol restrictions on patient selection, procedure performance or adjunctive therapy. Trial procedures are simplified and evolution in therapy can be accommodated. The principal disadvantages relate to a risk that the study may recruit a very diverse patient population managed with an experimental procedure that is subject to multiple variation.

Problems in the application of RCT methodology to trials of surgical/interventional procedures

- timing of study initiation
  - 'learning curve' effect
- blinding for outcome measure assessment
- evaluation of markedly different therapies
- recruitment of a representative population
- coping with changing treatment patterns
  - pragmatic trial design

Conclusions

There are a number of well-characterized limitations when classical drug trial methodology is applied to the assessment of procedures. Careful study design can overcome some issues but many studies will still involve the unblinded assessment of two (or more) very different treatment options. This presents special problems in patient recruitment and informed consent that can only be addressed in recruiting centers.

CHAPTER 3
Statistical principles in clinical trials

Ameet Bakhai, Duolao Wang & Marcus Flather

Introduction

Clinical trial design, analysis and interpretation rely upon statistical principles. All statistical tests make certain pre-specified assumptions about the data. For example, parametric statistics rely on the assumption that data have a 'normal' distribution. An understanding of these assumptions is important not only for the design and analysis of clinical trials, but also for the critical appraisal of completed trials. In this chapter some important statistical principles are described and their relevance to clinical trials discussed. At the end of the chapter a glossary of commonly used statistical terms is provided.

Descriptive statistics

Descriptive statistics are commonly used to present the baseline characteristics of a population enrolled in a clinical trial. Descriptive statistics include tabulation of results, calculation of averages (means), and minimum/maximum values (range) or standard deviations (spread). The mode is the most frequent observation, and the median is the middle of all the values when these are ranked in order. Descriptive statistics are an essential part of reporting the results of a study, but they do not provide comparisons within the data set, or between one data set and another.

The concept of statistical 'normality'

Systolic blood pressure measurements of 1000 subjects participating in a lifestyle survey are shown in **Figure 1**. The distribution of these blood pressures conforms to a bell-shaped curve or 'normal' distribution typical for common, continuous biological measurements. The curve has particular mathematical properties expressed by the equation shown with the curve. The normal distribution was described by the German mathematician Gauss (1777–1855), and is also called the 'Gaussian' distribution. The standard deviation helps to describe the spread of the observations. In a normal distribution, about 68% of all observations lie within one standard deviation either side of the mean, and about 95% of all observations lie within two standard deviations either side of the mean. Other distributions, which are skewed to one side or the other, are also possible. These distributions are not 'normal', and the median is usually a more useful parameter than the mean in representing the central location of these distributions.

The null hypothesis and the alternative hypothesis

To explain the null and alternative hypotheses, we can use an example of a study investigating a new treatment to reduce the mortality (death) rate after myocardial infarction. The simplest form of comparison is a two group, placebo-controlled randomized trial. One group receives the active treatment and the other receives a placebo. The traditional 'null' hypothesis (H_0) for this trial assumes that the effect of the active treatment on mortality after myocardial infarction is the same as that of the placebo. The 'alternative' hypothesis (H_1) assumes that there is a difference in the mortality rates between the active and placebo treatments.

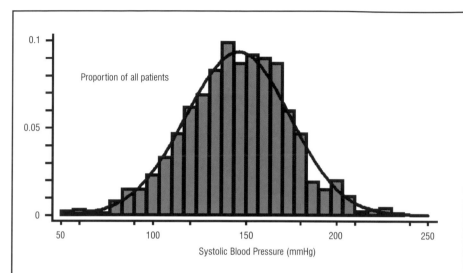

Equation:

$$f(x) = \frac{1}{\sigma\sqrt{2\pi}} \exp(\frac{-(x-\mu)^2}{2\sigma^2}), \sigma > 0, -\infty < \mu < \infty, -\infty < x < \infty$$

Description of the curve:

The curve of normal distribution has the following characteristics:

- The curve has a single peak at the center, this peak occurs at the mean (μ)
- The curve is symmetrical about the mean
- The curve never touches the horizontal axis
- The total area under the curve is equal to 1
- The width or shape of the curve is described by the variance (σ^2), the square root of which is the standard deviation (σ)

FIGURE 1. The normal distribution curve for blood pressures from 1000 patients

The results of the trial above may show:

1. That there is an apparent difference in mortality rates between the active and placebo treatment groups. In this case the null hypothesis (H_0) is rejected, and the alternative hypothesis (H_1) is accepted

2. That there is apparently no difference in treatment effects between the two groups. In this case the null hypothesis (H_0) is accepted

When making statistical comparisons between two groups of the trial, it is possible that there may be errors associated with these calculations, so that the effect seen may not completely reflect the true effect.

Alpha and beta (type I and type II) errors

- The alpha (type I) error occurs when the study finds a difference, but in truth none exists (a false positive). In this scenario the study findings support the alternative hypothesis but in truth the null hypothesis is correct. Usually the acceptable alpha error is set at 0.05, or 1 in 20. In other words, the likelihood of incorrectly accepting H_1 is 1 in 20 or less

- The beta (type II) error occurs when the study finds no difference, but in truth a difference does exist (a false negative). In this scenario the study findings support the null hypothesis, but in truth the alternative hypothesis is correct. The usual acceptable beta error is 0.20 or 1 in 5. In this case it is accepted that if a 'true' difference were present it would be detected 4 times out of 5

These errors are set at different levels because investigators have traditionally, and understandably, been more cautious about declaring false positives than false negatives. The stringency of each error can be varied according to circumstances. In some situations it may be more useful to assume that the alpha error is 0.01, or 1 in a 100, and the beta error is 0.1, or 1 in 10. These variations have an impact on sample size estimations, as discussed below.

How big should I make my trial?

In addition to the proposed alpha and beta errors, two further pieces of information are required to estimate the sample size: first, an estimate of the expected event rate in the control group of the trial (the group that is receiving standard care or placebo) is needed; second, an estimate of the likely reduction in event rates assuming the new treatment were to have a beneficial effect (for example, a 20% reduction in mortality). These estimates are usually based on previous studies (trials or registries), experience and some guesswork. Sometimes a range of treatment differences may be used. For example, if only one previous small study is available, using the range of the mean effect from that study ('standard error of the mean') may be more useful in determining the correct sample size (say 10–30% reduction). One can understand that estimating sample size can be an inexact science! Nevertheless a carefully constructed sample size estimate is important for clinical trials, especially for large trials where the sample size has important effects on the resources required.

A common term used when describing the sample size of a trial is 'power'. Power refers to the ability of a particular sample size to detect the 'true' difference. Power is determined from 1 minus the beta error and is usually set at 0.8 (or 80%). To increase the power of a trial more patients would be required. It should be noted that sample size is not a linear function. Thus, to detect a proportional difference of 15% will take approximately four times as many patients as to detect a difference of 30% if all other assumptions remain equal. In large clinical trials the alpha and/or beta errors are often more stringent than the standard 0.05 and 0.2. A range of sample

---

Example calculation of sample size for a study

The sample size for a hypothetical study can be estimated as follows:

- Expected event rate at 30 days = 50% (The first probability or P_1)
- Expected proportional risk reduction with new treatment = 20%:
  i.e. 50% reduced to 40% (The second probability or P_2)
- $P=(P_1+P_2)/2$
- Alpha error set at 0.05 (α), this gives a significance threshold level of 5%
- Beta error set at 0.2 (β), this gives at least 80% power to detect the expected risk reduction
- Z ($\alpha/2$) and Z (β) are constants from the standard normal distribution depending on the values of α and β

Given the above parameters, the following formula can be used to calculate the sample size required in each treatment arm:

$$n = \frac{[Z(\alpha/2)\sqrt{2P(1-P)} + z(\beta)\sqrt{P_1(1-P_1) + P_2(1-P_2)}]^2}{(P_1-P_2)^2}$$

From these conditions, the following parameters are derived:
$P_1=0.50$, $P_2=0.40$, $P=(0.50+0.40)/2=0.45$, $z(\alpha/2)=1.96$, $z(\beta)=0.842$

Using the formula for the sample size calculation:

$$n = \frac{[1.96\sqrt{2*0.45(1-0.45)} + 0.842\sqrt{0.50(1-0.50) + 0.40(1-0.40)}]^2}{(0.50-0.40)^2} = 388$$

(* denotes the multiplication sign)

Therefore a sample size of 388 patients per arm is required to obtain an 80% power for detection of a difference of 20% between the two treatment groups.

sizes, based on variations of the errors and expected probabilities, should be considered for most trials, and a balance struck between power and available resources.

Classification of data

Results obtained in a clinical trial can be expressed in different ways. Measurement of blood pressure, weight, height, plasma cholesterol, serum creatinine and left ventricular ejection fraction are examples of 'continuous' variables. Continuous variables can be expressed at different levels of precision depending on the scale of the measurement methods (for example centimeters or millimeters). In contrast, measurement of death, hospital admission, strokes and myocardial infarctions are examples of 'dichotomous' or 'binary' variables. Dichotomous variables (also called 'categorical' variables) have only two possible outcomes. Thus in a trial evaluating the effects of a new treatment on mortality, patients can be classified as having one of two conditions: either dead or alive. Most measurements in clinical trials can be classified as continuous or dichotomous.

Other ways of expressing measurements include assigning grades or 'ranks'. For example, when asked 'Do you feel depressed?' a patient may be asked to select the most appropriate answer from the following: 'never, sometimes, often, always'. The patient's response has four possible categories that can be ranked from mild to severe. Statistical assumptions for these data are different from those for numerical data. An alternative approach to the reporting of continuous variables is to convert the continuous data into categorical data. This is done by dividing the patients into subgroups of either equal size or by chosen limits for each subgroup. The types of data recorded will determine the appropriate statistical tests required.

Comparison of continuous variables

The most commonly used statistical test for the comparison of results (continuous variables) from two sample populations is the 't' test. The 't' test compares the means of two sets of continuous variables and expresses the probability that any differences are due to the play of chance (i.e. that the null hypothesis is supported), or may be 'real' (i.e. that the alternative hypothesis is supported). This probability is often calculated from a 't' value.

Example of a comparison of continuous variables – 't' test

An example calculation in a study to evaluate the effects of a treatment to reduce blood pressure is given. A trial comparing the effect of an anti-hypertensive therapy against placebo was set up. The results of the two groups of patients were as follows:

Results of blood pressures

- In the control group of 548 patients the mean systolic blood pressure was 150.22 with a standard deviation of 27.12 mmHg

- In the treatment group of 550 patients the mean systolic blood pressure was 146.78 with a standard deviation of 28.32 mmHg

Using these data the 't' test can be calculated in the following manner:
Suppose two groups of sizes n_1 and n_2 have blood pressure results with means $\bar{x}_1$ and $\bar{x}_2$ and standard deviations s_1 and s_2, respectively. Then the efficacy of the treatment, as compared to placebo, can be examined by testing the following hypotheses:

$$H_0 : \mu_1 = \mu_2$$
$$H_1 : \mu_1 \neq \mu_2$$

The t statistic for the above test is given by $t = \dfrac{\bar{x}_1 - \bar{x}_2}{\sqrt{\dfrac{(n_1 - 1)s_1^2 + (n_2 - 1)s_2^2}{n_1 + n_2 - 2}} \sqrt{\dfrac{1}{n_1} + \dfrac{1}{n_2}}}$

Therefore the null hypothesis can be rejected ($H_0 : \mu_1 = \mu_2$) at the α level of significance if $|t| \geq t(\alpha/2, n_1 + n_2 - 2)$, where $t(\alpha/2, n_1 + n_2 - 2)$ is the upper $(\alpha/2)$th percentile of the t-distribution with $n_1 + n_2 - 2$ degrees of freedom.

In this case, we have $n_1 = 548$, $n_2 = 550$, $\bar{x}_1 = 150.22$, $\bar{x}_2 = 146.78$, $s_1 = 27.12$, $s_2 = 28.32$ Substituting the above sample statistics into the 't' test formula, we obtain t = 2.0555 which equates to a probability of 0.040 that the two populations are the same.

This implies that there is a statistically significant difference in the systolic blood pressures between the two treatment groups. In other words the drug appears to reduce systolic blood pressure compared to placebo and the result has a low likelihood of arising by chance.

Statistical approaches to comparisons of dichotomous variables

The most common statistical approaches for the randomized comparison of two groups, using a dichotomous outcome such as death, are the chi-squared (χ^2) test and the Fisher exact test. The chi-squared test involves determining the expected number of deaths in the treatment and placebo arms and then comparing these to the observed number. The test statistic used to assess these differences in death rate can be expressed as

$$\chi^2 = \sum \frac{(O - E)^2}{E}$$

where O represents the observed frequencies and E the expected frequencies in each treatment arm. Under the null hypothesis of no difference, chi-squared has a distribution with approximately 1 degree of freedom. The Fisher exact test consists of evaluating the sum of probabilities associated with the observed frequencies table and all possible two-by-two tables that have the same row and column totals as the observed data. When sample size is large, a test of the difference between two proportions also uses a normally distributed test statistic Z, which can be easily calculated by hand.

Example of a comparison of dichotomous variables – 'Z' test

The results of a trial to evaluate a treatment to reduce the rate of death after myocardial infarction might have the following results:

- Group 1 (treatment)   110 deaths out of a total of 2045 patients
- Group 2 (placebo)   165 deaths out of a total of 2022 patients

Statistical inference of binary data from a parallel two-group trial involves testing the hypotheses regarding the difference in proportions with a 'yes' response between the treatment and the placebo group. This can be expressed as

$$H_0 : \pi_1 = \pi_2$$
$$H_1 : \pi_1 \neq \pi_2$$

The statistic for the above test is given by

$$Z = \frac{\hat{p}_1 - \hat{p}_2}{\sqrt{\hat{p}_p(1 - \hat{p}_p)(1/n_1 + 1/n_2)}}$$

Where n_1 and n_2 are the sample sizes (2045 and 2022), x_1 and x_2 the number of events in the two groups (110 and 165) respectively and $\hat{p}_1 = \frac{x_1}{n_1}(= 110/2045 = 0.054)$

$\hat{p}_2 = \frac{x_2}{n_2}(= 165/2022 = 0.082)$ and $\hat{p}_p = \frac{x_1 + x_2}{n_1 + n_2}(= [(110+165)/(2045+2022)] = 0.068)$.

Therefore the null hypothesis can be rejected ($H_0 : \pi_1 = \pi_2$) at the α level of significance if $|Z| \geq Z(\alpha/2)$, where $Z(\alpha/2)$ is the upper $(\alpha/2)$th percentile of the standard normal distribution.

In this case $Z = -3.548$ which equates to a probability of p=0.0004.

This suggests that patients in the treatment group have a statistically significant lower death rate than patients in the placebo group.

Other statistical tests and terminology

A glossary of terms appended to this chapter covers many of the statistical terms that the reader may encounter in journal articles. Recommendations for further reading to explore these terms in more detail are provided at the end of the chapter.

Conclusions

Statistical assumptions and methods are essential in the design, conduct and analysis of clinical trials. An analysis plan summarising the outcome measures and how they will be compared should be an integral part of all study protocols. This plan should be expanded and finalized prior to analysing the data. Randomized studies require substantial resources, and it makes sense to obtain the best advice before using these resources. The advice of a statistician with experience in medical research should be obtained from the design stage through to the completion and analysis phases of all trials.

GLOSSARY OF COMMONLY USED STATISTICAL TERMS

CONFIDENCE INTERVALS

A range of values within which the 'true' population mean is likely to lie. Usually 95% confidence limits are quoted which implies there is 95% confidence in the statement that the 'true' population mean will lie somewhere between the upper and lower limits.

CORRELATION COEFFICIENT (r)

A measure of the linear association between two continuous variables. The correlation coefficient varies between -1.0 and +1.0. The closer it is to 0, the weaker the association. When both variables go in the same direction (example: height and weight), r has a positive value between 0 and 1.0 depending on the strength of the relationship. When the variables go in opposite directions (example: left ventricular function and life-span), r has a negative value between 0 and -1.0 depending on the strength of this inverse relationship. The Spearman rank correlation coefficient is one example of a correlation coefficient. It is used when it is not convenient or possible to give actual values to variables, but only to assign a rank order (quartiles or subgroups) to instances of each variable.

END-POINTS/OUTCOME EVENTS

Outcomes may be based on safety, efficacy or another trial objective (such as radiation exposure) and should be clearly defined in the protocol. Outcomes or endpoints may occur in two situations:

1. When a patient has a pre-specified protocol outcome such as a heart attack or death, they have reached an end-point for the study

2. When the patient reaches completion of a trial without any adverse outcomes

INTENTION-TO-TREAT ANALYSIS

A method of data analysis on the basis of the intention to treat a subject (i.e., the planned treatment regimen) rather than the actual treatment regimen given. It has the consequence that subjects allocated to a treatment group should be followed up, assessed and analysed as members of that group regardless of their compliance with therapy or the protocol, or whether they crossed over later to the other treatment group.

MULTIVARIATE/UNIVARIATE ANALYSIS

'Variates' refers to the term variable or parameter. A univariate analysis examines the association between a single variable and an adverse outcome variable. For example, age and occurrence of stroke. The influence (likelihood of outcome) of each variable is presented as a mean value and confidence intervals. In univariate analysis each factor is looked at separately so that the influence may be magnified. In a multivariate analysis, the influence of each variable is determined, taking into account the influence of other variables included in the analysis. The analysis can be undertaken to determine the association between several risk factors, for example; age, sex, systolic blood pressure and cholesterol level, and the outcome incidence of stroke. Multivariate analysis may help to reduce the confounding effects of other variables or co-variates but involves more complex statistics than univariate analyses.

ODDS RATIO (OR) and RELATIVE RISK (or RISK RATIO, RR)

These terms describe the probability of an outcome by comparing two groups. The relative risk (RR) is the ratio of the probability of disease among those exposed compared to the probability of disease among those unexposed. The odds ratio (OR) is the ratio of patients with and without disease in the two comparison groups. If the death rates in the treatment and control arms of a randomized study

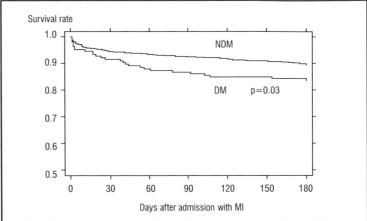

In this diagram we can see that a larger proportion of non-diabetic patients (0.9) are alive at 180 days after an admission with an MI than diabetic patients (0.83, p=0.03)

FIGURE 2. Example of a Kaplan-Meier curve examining the rates of death over time, after admission with a myocardial infarction (MI) for patients with and without diabetes mellitus (DM)

Suggested further reading

Altman DG. *Practical Statistics for Medical Research*. Chapman and Hall. 1999.
Chow SC. *Encyclopedia of Biopharmaceutical Statistics*. Marcel Dekker, Inc. 2000.
Chow SC, Liu JP. *Design and Analysis of Clinical Trials: Concepts and Methodologies*. John Wiley. 1998.
Pocock SJ. *Clinical Trials: A Practical Approach*. Wiley. 1983.
Everitt BS, Pickles A. *Statistical Aspects of the Design and Analysis of Clinical Trials*. Imperial College Press. 1999.
Sterne JAC, Smith GD. Sifting the evidence - what's wrong with significance tests? *Br Med J* 2001;**322**:226–31.

CHAPTER 4

Regulatory and ethical issues in clinical trials

Hazel Aston, Jean Booth & Marrianne Stuteville

Regulatory issues

Why are regulatory authorities involved in clinical trials?

The development and sale of drugs and devices for human use is supervised by regulatory authorities appointed by Governments to ensure that products are safe, effective for their intended use, and that all aspects of development, manufacturing and clinical investigation conform to agreed quality standards. The necessity for drug safety control was highlighted by human tragedy with disasters caused by use of sulfanilamide (high mortality rate) in the USA in 1937 and thalidomide (phocomelia) in Europe and Australia in the 1960s.

What are the phases of clinical trial activity?

Appropriate regulation of clinical trials requires some formalization of trial procedures. The Food and Drug Administration (FDA) first described the four 'phases' for development of a new drug in humans. This terminology is now widely accepted throughout the pharmaceutical industry. The phases are listed in **Table 1**.

Phase I	• First investigation of a new drug in humans (often called 'first into man' studies) • Investigation of the pharmacokinetics and the pharmacologic effects of a drug, including dose-response and side effects • Small numbers of subjects, usually healthy volunteers
Phase II	• Information gained in Phase I is used to design Phase II studies • Closely controlled and monitored studies conducted in small numbers of patients (<100) • Provides preliminary efficacy and safety data
Phase III	• Demonstrates the efficacy and safety of a drug • Involves hundreds or thousands of patients • Phase IIIb studies investigate new indications for already licensed drugs
Phase IV	• Surveillance in many thousands of patients to identify less common adverse effects • Post-marketing studies to investigate the use of a drug in special populations of patients

TABLE 1. Phase I–IV development of a new drug

Clinical studies can also be classified according to the objective of the study as follows:

• Human pharmacology
• Therapeutic exploratory
• Therapeutic confirmatory
• Therapeutic use

The objective defined studies listed above may be performed at different temporal phases (I–IV) of drug development. For example, human pharmacology studies are usually carried out during Phase I of drug development but may also be performed following Phase III studies to investigate adverse events observed at this stage of development. Further information is contained within the International Conference on Harmonisation (ICH) Guideline E8, General Considerations for Clinical Trials. Copies of this and other ICH guidelines can be downloaded from the ICH web site (see 'Useful web sites' at the end of this chapter).

Who regulates the development and sale of pharmaceutical products and what procedures do they impose?

Most countries take measures to regulate the development and marketing of medicinal products for human use. The USA, European Union (EU) and Japan represent the major markets for pharmaceutical products. The regulatory authorities in each of these areas are listed in **Table 2**.

	USA	EU	Japan
Regulatory body	Food and Drug Administration (FDA)	The European Agency for the Evaluation of Medicinal Products (EMEA) represents all European member states	Ministry of Health and Welfare (MHW)
Advisory/ administrative bodies	Center for Drug Evaluation and Research (CDER)	The Committee for Proprietary Medicinal Products (CPMP) acts as a scientific advisory body to the EMEA	Central Pharmaceutical Affairs Council (CPAC) and the Pharmaceutical and Medical Device Evaluation Centre (PMDEC)
Key regulations	Food, Drug and Cosmetic Act, 1938. Code of Federal Regulations (CFR) title 21	Directive 65/65/European Economic Community (EEC), 1965	The Pharmaceutical Affairs Law, 1960

TABLE 2. Regulatory authorities for pharmaceutical products in the USA, EU and Japan

The regulatory procedures and key regulations that apply in the USA and EU are listed in **Table 3**. Separate bodies such as the Center for Biologics Evaluation and Research (CBER) and the Center for Devices and Radiological Health (CDRH) in the USA control clinical trials and marketing authorizations for biologics and biotechnology products and medical devices, respectively.

Application for clinical trials to proceed

USA	EU
• an Investigational New Drug (IND) application must be submitted to the FDA	• applications are submitted to the National regulatory authority of individual EC Member States (MS)
• the submission permits shipment of investigational products across state lines	• procedures vary from one country to another and at different phases of the clinical trial process
• the FDA has 30 days to review the IND application	• Germany, France and Portugal require notification for all stages of clinical trials
• the application can be put on 'clinical hold' if the FDA judges that it is not safe to proceed	• the UK imposes no regulatory steps for Phase I studies but must grant authorization for Phase II–IV clinical trials to proceed

TABLE 3. Regulatory procedures in the USA and EU

Application for a marketing authorization (MA)

USA

- a New Drug Application (NDA) must be submitted to the FDA
- the FDA reviews the dossier to ensure that the drug is effective and safe for its intended purpose
- complete data as outlined in the 'Notice to Applicants', including CRF data, must be submitted
- one of nine Offices for Drug Evaluation (ODE), each one with responsibility for specific therapeutic areas, evaluates the data including a statistical analysis of raw data and factory and laboratory inspections to validate the submission
- the FDA will issue a refusal to file notice for all NDA submissions that contain insufficient information to perform a review
- the review of the submission takes 6 or 12 months depending on whether it is judged to be a priority or standard application
- following the review, the FDA will issue an action letter to say that the NDA is approved, approvable (stating the deficiencies in the application) or not approvable

EU

Three procedures exist:

1. national application to an individual MS

2. centralized procedure

- an application is submitted to the European Medicines Evaluation Agency (EMEA) for biotechnology or high tech products
- the EMEA acts as an administrative body
- a rapporteur from one of the 15 EC MS assesses the application and reports to the Committee for Proprietary Medicinal Products (CPMP)
- the CPMP, comprised of two representatives from each of the 15 MS, reviews the assessment report and permits or refuses authorization
- approval permits sale of the drug in all 15 MS

3. decentralized (mutual recognition) procedure.

- for products that do not fit into the centralized procedure
- once approval is obtained in one MS an applicant can request mutual recognition of this reference authorization by all or some of the other MS

Commitments after a marketing authorization (MA) has been granted

USA

- a report must be submitted annually
- Medwatch performs pharmacovigilance on behalf of the FDA
- serious adverse reactions where there is a suspected association with the medicinal product or instances where the quality, safety or performance of a product is impaired can be reported to Medwatch either directly or via the pharmaceutical sponsor

EU

- sponsors are required to notify the regulatory authority of minor changes to an MA and to seek approval for any major changes
- variations to an MA may occur as a result of adverse drug reactions, because of a change in manufacturing process or to comply with new directives and guidelines
- an application for renewal of an MA should be submitted five years after the MA was first granted and every five years thereafter

Regulations versus guidelines

Regulations, such as those presented in **Table 2**, have legal status, are enforceable by law and are therefore a mandatory requirement. Guidelines also exist and although highly recommended and often enforced by commercial sponsors of trials, they are not legally binding. The well-established ICH Good Clinical Practice (GCP) guideline is a key document influencing the conduct of clinical trials and will be discussed in more detail below. Other guidelines deal with different aspects of drug development and production and include ICH Good Laboratory Practice (GLP) and Good Manufacturing Practice (GMP) guidelines.

What is the ICH?

The International Conference on Harmonisation of Technical Requirements for Registration of Pharmaceuticals for Human Use is a joint initiative involving regulators and the pharmaceutical industry. Six parties are directly involved plus observers and the ICH secretariat.

The six members of the ICH are:

- European Commission – European Union (EU)
- European Federation of Pharmaceutical Industries' Associations (EFPIA)
- Ministry of Health and Welfare, Japan (MHW)
- Japan Pharmaceutical Manufacturers Association (JPMA)
- USA Food and Drug Administration (FDA)
- Pharmaceutical Research and Manufacturers of America (PhRMA)

What is the ICH GCP guideline?

The ICH GCP guideline is an international ethical and scientific quality standard for the design, conduct, recording and reporting of trials in human subjects. It was developed to protect the rights, safety and well being of trial subjects, based on the Declaration of Helsinki, and to assure the credibility of clinical trials. The guideline provides a unified standard for the EU, Japan and the USA to facilitate mutual acceptance of clinical data by regulatory authorities in these jurisdictions.

The subject areas covered by the guideline are:

- glossary
- principles
- Institutional Review Board/Independent Ethics Committee (IRB/IEC)

- the investigator
- the sponsor
- clinical trial protocol and protocol amendments
- Investigators' brochure
- essential documents for the conduct of a clinical trial (e.g. the investigator brochure, trial protocol and ethical committee approval)

What are the responsibilities of the investigator according to the ICH GCP guideline?

The responsibilities of the investigator are outlined in detail in section 4 of the ICH GCP guideline. The main elements are:

- to protect the rights, safety and welfare of individuals who have agreed to participate in the trial
- to ensure informed consent is obtained for all patients participating in the trial
- to ensure that the investigation is conducted according to the protocol, case report forms and applicable regulations
- to ensure drugs or medical devices are stored appropriately and are only used for the purpose of the study. The investigator is accountable for all investigational products
- to identify staff who are appropriately trained for their role in the clinical trial and provide documentation of their qualifications
- to ensure correct documentation in case report forms and patient hospital records to enable source data verification
- to be available for monitoring visits and to permit the trial monitors access to source data
- to store the study data for the appropriate time required by regulations for that individual study

- to report adverse events according to the regulatory guidelines for the individual study

The principles of ICH GCP may be applied to **any** clinical research investigation that may have an impact on the safety and well being of human subjects.

What are clinical trial audits?

The ICH GCP guideline defines an audit as 'a systematic and independent examination of trial-related activities and documents.' The aim is to ensure that trials are conducted in accordance with the trial protocol, the sponsor's standard operating procedures (SOPs) and all applicable guidelines and regulatory requirements.

Clinical trial audits are performed by regulatory authorities, trial sponsors or organizations nominated by the trial sponsor (**Figure 1**). The regulatory authorities in the USA and EU perform audits of the sponsor, drug development facilities, manufacturing plants and study sites. These audits may be extensive and assessors may spend several days at a site. Study sites are given advance notification that an audit will be conducted. Negative audit findings vary in severity from deficiencies in essential trial documentation that can be easily rectified, to errors in consent procedures and investigator fraud. Serious discrepancies may lead to termination of a trial at a study site or legal proceedings against an investigator.

Why do I need to know about regulatory issues?

Usually, investigators do not need a detailed knowledge of regulatory affairs in order to participate in a clinical trial. Industrial sponsors have regulatory affairs departments to ensure that they comply with the current regulations and guidelines, as mistakes may adversely affect applications for regulatory approval. Although the study sponsor ensures that

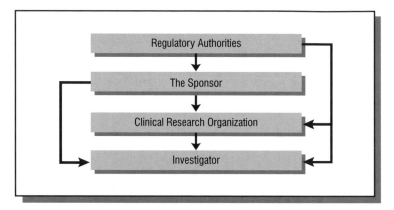

FIGURE 1. Potential audits within a clinical trial

all necessary documentation is completed and submitted to the appropriate regulatory body, the regulatory process may impose a substantial workload on the study sites. Investigators must be meticulous about data quality, the administration of all trial documentation and adherence to the trial protocol and consent procedures in order to fulfill their responsibilities according to the ICH GCP guideline.

Ethics in clinical research

The Declaration of Helsinki forms the ethical basis for all clinical research involving human subjects. The World Medical Association adopted the declaration in 1964 but there have been subsequent amendments, the most recent in October 2000. A copy of the declaration can be downloaded from the UK Multi-Centre Research Ethics Committee (MREC) web site (see 'Useful web sites' at end of chapter).

What is the role of an ethics committee?

An ethics committee is an independent body of medical professionals and lay members. The responsibility of an ethics committee is to ensure that the safety, well being and human rights of subjects participating in a clinical trial are protected. Ethics committees review the protocol and consent forms to ensure that the trial is justified, safe and that patients are properly informed. All research involving human subjects should be referred to the local Institutional Review Board (IRB) or Independent Ethics Committee (IEC).

The legal status, constitution and responsibilities of ethics committees may differ from country to country. The ICH GCP guideline recommends that an IRB/IEC should comprise at least five members, at least one of which should have a primary area of interest in a non-scientific area, and at least one of which should be independent of the institution or trial site.

According to the ICH GCP guideline, the responsibilities of IRBs/IECs are:

- to review and process an application for ethical approval of a research protocol within a reasonable time
- to consider the qualifications of the investigator
- to review each ongoing trial at an institution
- to recommend modifications to the patient information and consent sheet, where appropriate
- to review payments to trial subjects
- to determine that, where necessary, the trial protocol addresses ethical concerns for consent by a subject's legal representative and studies where prior consent is not possible
- to perform its duties in accordance with written operating procedures
- to retain all relevant records for at least three years after completion of a trial

What is the system of ethical review?
The procedures for ethical approval of a trial protocol vary from country to country and from institution to institution.

Many countries in Europe now have a two-tiered system of ethics review, e.g. the MREC and the Local Research Ethics Committee (LREC) system in the UK. Within this system, the MREC reviews a trial protocol if five or more LREC geographical boundaries are involved in a trial. MREC approval is submitted to the LREC at each study site along with the trial protocol and all other supporting documentation. The LREC's primary concerns are local issues such as the qualifications of the local researcher and the patient information and consent form.

What is informed consent?

Informed consent is the process by which a subject voluntarily confirms his or her willingness to participate in a clinical trial. Prior to giving consent, the subject must be informed of all aspects of the trial including the risks and benefits of taking part. The subject should be informed of their rights as outlined in the Declaration of Helsinki. Informed consent must be documented by means of a written consent form. A copy of the consent form, signed and dated by the subject and the investigator, should be given to the subject or their legal representative.

What is required for a patient information and consent form?

In multicenter studies the patient information and consent form is usually distributed to centers for submission to the local IEC/IRB. Items for inclusion in the information and consent form have been defined by ICH and are listed in section 4 of the ICH GCP guideline. Although these items are generally recognized by most bodies as being desirable to include in the patient information sheet, there may be different national or local requirements that need to be considered when producing a patient information and consent form. According to the ICH GCP guideline the main elements which should be included are:

- explanation of the research that is being performed
- explanation of the aim of the trial, the proposed treatment and description of procedures
- anticipated duration of the trial and number of subjects to be included
- the potential benefits to the subject (if there are no potential benefits to the individual participating in the trial this must be made clear)
- a statement of any potential risks or discomfort
- any alternative therapies
- a statement of randomization, if used in the trial
- any payments or anticipated expenses for participating in the trial
- compensation available in the event of trial-related injury
- a statement that participation is voluntary and that the subject may withdraw at any time
- a statement that all information pertaining to the trial is confidential and will be presented anonymously

Summary

- The responsibility of a regulatory authority is to ensure that products are safe, effective for their intended use, and that all aspects of development, manufacturing and clinical investigation conform to agreed quality standards
- The responsibility of an ethics committee is to ensure that the safety, well being and human rights of subjects participating in a clinical trial are protected

Regulatory affairs and medical ethics are extensive and continually evolving subjects with changes in guidelines and regulatory requirements being frequently implemented. Consequently, it is only possible to provide an overview of

Scientific aspects

What question does the trial address?

It is important to determine that the trial addresses a question of clinical and scientific relevance. Some trials permit a commercial sponsor to apply for an extension to the marketing authorization of an investigational product but do little to improve our understanding of disease and therapeutics. The same question is sometimes addressed many times by different companies and some proposals may be redundant as the information is readily available.

Will the study be published and who will write the manuscript? What will happen if the study demonstrates a negative finding?

Is the study likely to achieve its goals?

Other chapters of this handbook discuss clinical trial design and statistical issues and should permit an investigator to assess whether a protocol is likely to confirm or refute a trial's hypothesis. An important consideration for investigators is whether the sample size stated in the protocol can be enrolled in the timeframe allowed. Also, the requirements for follow-up of patients must be considered; e.g. the duration and frequency of follow-up, and the data to be collected.

What population of patients will the trial enroll?

Eligibility criteria must be carefully assessed; it is easy to overestimate the number of patients at a study site who might be eligible for a trial. Some study sites keep records of admissions to combat this problem. More experienced study sites can often use information from previous trials that had similar eligibility criteria as a guide.

Investigators should be confident that sufficient eligible patients will be recruited for the study. A useful exercise is to perform a survey of potentially eligible patients over 2–4 weeks. This will provide a guide to estimated recruitment rates.

What impact will the trial have on patients?

This is perhaps one of the most important questions. An investigator's primary obligation is to protect the welfare of his/her patients. An investigator should consider how much time the patient will have to devote to the study and any compensation the patient may receive. Also, will patients be required to have investigations that would not be considered part of routine care and, if so, will they be painful or put the patient at additional risk? Ethics committees pay particular attention to these issues when reviewing a trial protocol.

How will the data be collected and recorded?

Data collection is a time-consuming task, especially if case report forms ask for vast amounts of data, much of which may contribute little to the study results. How will the data be amassed and recorded, and what impact will this have on the study coordinator? Procedures for processing adverse events may be very time-consuming and this may not be clear at the outset of the trial.

What staff will be required to perform the trial?

Before committing to participation in a clinical trial, it is essential to ensure that the department and institution have staff available to run the trial and that these people are sufficiently experienced in clinical trials (**Table 1**). This is particularly true of the study coordinator and any sub-investigators who will be assigned the task of running the trial on a day-to-day basis. Curricula vitae are usually requested by the study sponsor because it is a requirement of the International Conference on Harmonisation Good Clinical Practice (ICH GCP) guideline that staff are appropriately qualified. It is important to assess the amount of time required for patient enrollment, data collection and follow-up, and to consider whether study staff will have time to fulfill these obligations.

Important notes

When calculating the staff costs, it is important to consider the following questions:

- How many staff will be needed to fulfill the requirements of the protocol?
- What are the salary levels of people identified?
- What proportion of their time will be spent on the study?

It is important to be realistic about your answers. If the level of remuneration is such that staff costs will not be completely covered it is best to know this in advance.

Staff member	Key responsibilities
Sub-investigator It is essential to appoint a medically qualified sub-investigator	Responsibilities include: • obtaining consent from patients • provision of medical advice in relation to eligibility criteria, concomitant treatments or other clinical issues
Study coordinator/Nurse Perhaps the most important member of the clinical trials team, the study coordinator is *involved at all stages of a trial*	Responsibilities include: • ensuring that all essential documents are obtained from the sponsor and submitted for institutional and ethical review • screening for eligible patients • randomizing patients into a study • recording data on case report forms and responding to data queries • completing and submitting adverse event reports within the timelines specified in the protocol • liaising with staff in other departments to ensure that the trial runs smoothly and that it is advertised and understood within the institution • ensuring that all data are appropriately archived in accordance with the procedures set by the trial sponsor at study close-out • ensuring that all relevant documentation is available at monitoring and audit visits
Pharmacist Some institutions have dedicated clinical trials pharmacists, especially where there are many trials across a number of *therapeutic areas*	Responsibilities include: • storage and disposal of investigational products (there may be special rules concerning the storage and disposal of investigational products) • dispensing (often requires special protocols)
Laboratory staff Trials usually require that a patient has a number of *clinical investigations*	Responsibilities include: • carrying out routine measurements • special procedures for the purpose of the trial • processing and short-term storage of blood samples

TABLE 1. Staffing requirements

Financial aspects

Payments to study sites vary from study to study but the principles applied when reaching a decision to participate in a trial should remain the same.

What will the local costs be?

Most institutions now have a specific department, or an appointed external group, to review studies and ensure that local health service resources are not being used inappropriately to subsidize research. Prior to submitting a study for review by such groups, investigators should perform a financial review themselves and ideally develop a local budget. Local costs are usually predictable and are outlined in **Table 2**. However, it is important to remember that there may be many 'hidden' costs in running trials including costs of drug storage, ethics committee review and provision of laboratory certificates. If specimens are to be sent to a central laboratory, ensure that costs of local processing, storage and shipping are covered.

Is the payment schedule optimal?

Investigators should also consider the structure of the payment schedule. Most research studies pay a set amount of money per patient recruited, but the timing of such payments can vary. Possible payment schedules are:

- one payment per patient when the patient is recruited
- one payment per patient once certain pre-specified data have been declared 'clean', i.e. free from omissions or inaccuracies, and hence appropriate for statistical analysis
- one payment per patient at the time that the entire dataset has been received and declared 'clean'
- a structured payment schedule whereby set amounts are paid at recruitment, for the receipt of data from various follow-up visits and at the time that the entire dataset has been declared 'clean'

Whilst the first of these methods has obvious benefits to the investigator, it is becoming increasingly rare. As sponsors/trial coordinators need to ensure the quality and completeness of the data collected on all patients it is more usual for payment to follow successful collection of all necessary data. Other criteria may apply, e.g. payments may only be made if the patients enrolled fulfill all of the study's eligibility criteria.

The investigator should make sure that all eventualities have been considered when agreeing to undertake a study where the payments are based upon receipt of 'clean' data and/or are tied to follow-up visits. They can do this by ensuring that they have asked the following questions.

- *Are the local personnel sufficiently skilled/motivated such that all case record form pages and related data queries can be completed accurately and in a timely manner?*

Investigators must be aware that there is a potential for payments to be withheld if this is not the case.

- Is *the study patient-friendly?*

Will there be a high percentage of patients who choose to discontinue study treatment or refuse to attend for follow-up visits? Investigators should be able to answer these questions from past research experience. If payments are dependent on patient follow-up, then it is vital that these follow-ups take place. Also, contracts should be examined to ascertain what will happen in circumstances that are beyond the control of the investigator, e.g. the death of a patient.

• *Can contingency arrangements be made?*

Many protocols are amended in one way or another during the course of the study, and extension to recruitment periods is a real possibility. Investigators should be realistic in the financial planning of a project whilst ensuring that all costs are adequately covered by the contract.

Voice of experience

With each new research project, it will become easier to answer accurately the questions outlined above. Investigators are advised to keep complete records of trial income and expenditure. This effort will be valuable in assessing the financial implications of future research projects.

To participate or not to participate? That is the question!

Investigators usually choose to take part in a research study because they appreciate the scientific or clinical importance of the question. As such, they may be willing to subsidize research that is not adequately funded. It is less usual, but equally possible, that they may decide to participate simply because they feel that the study is well-funded.

Area/Department	Key responsibilities
Fees for laboratory and other clinical investigations	When tests are required, the following questions should be asked: • Are the tests part of routine care for the patient? (As such, these would represent no additional cost.) • If not, is additional funding provided for their conduct? • If funding for these tests is not specifically mentioned as part of the payment schedule, will the proposed remuneration cover their cost?
Pharmacy	Pharmacy costs will arise from provision of the following services: • set-up • dispensing • unblinding • out of hours assistance
IRB: Institutional Review Board; IEC: Independent Ethics Committee	Institutional Review Board fees vary from institution to institution and from study to study depending on the funding source. If these are not directly paid by the study sponsor then it is important to make provision for these from the payment received.
General equipment costs	It may be necessary to provide some or all of the following: • a dedicated fax machine • telephones, computers and office furniture for study personnel • facilities for storage (Clinical trials generate large quantities of paperwork, all of which must be archived in facilities that meet regulatory guidelines. Some institutions may not have sufficient space for this and it could, therefore, be necessary to pay for external archiving of study documentation.)
Special equipment	Upon review of the trial protocol, it may become apparent that some special analytical or laboratory equipment is needed. In this situation, the following questions should be addressed: • Does the institution already own this equipment? • If not, is additional funding available specifically for the equipment? • If not, will the proposed remuneration cover the costs of the equipment?
Staff training	This is a hidden cost that is often overlooked when evaluating the cost implications of a research project. Whilst for some studies this is a minimal cost, other studies may necessitate the involvement of many personnel all of whom may have differing levels of knowledge about the study area. If this is the case, investigators should be aware of the additional salary costs arising from ensuring that all staff are adequately trained.

TABLE 2. Local cost considerations

CHAPTER 6
Participating in multicenter clinical trials

Belinda Lees, Rebecca Mister & Ian Barnes

Introduction

Whilst many of the start-up activities are identical for both single-center and multicenter clinical trials, it is important to note that there may be particular issues regarding participation in a multicenter trial. A multicenter clinical trial usually involves a coordinating center with whom you will be required to liaise at each stage of the trial. The coordinating center will have specific procedures for enrolling and (where applicable) randomizing patients, performing any study-related measurements, recording data and reporting any adverse events. As a participant in a multicenter clinical trial you will be required to follow the protocol set down by the coordinating center and, therefore, you must ensure that the protocol is appropriate to your center.

Investigator meetings

Most multicenter trials have meetings for trial participants. These meetings usually take place at the start of the trial (to discuss the protocol and practical considerations of the trial), during the trial (to monitor progress and problems) and at the end of the trial (to present and discuss results). Investigator meetings are a good way to find out more about the trial and meet other participants.

	Main responsibilities
Coordinating center The academic group, industry sponsor or Contract Research Organization that takes responsibility for the initiation and management of the trial	• the coordinating center will be your point of contact for all trial-related matters including protocol issues, recruitment and data management
Principal and local investigators	• the principal investigator is usually an expert in the field and takes overall responsibility for the trial • each center will also have a local investigator who takes responsibility for the study at their site • the local investigator will often appoint a study coordinator or research nurse to assist in performing the study
Steering Committee Members usually include the main investigators, and other key people who take responsibility for the scientific integrity of the study	• the Steering Committee should meet prior to recruitment for the study to agree on the final protocol, then at regular intervals during the study to monitor progress, and finally at the end of the study to review the results
Data Safety and Monitoring Committee Members of the DSMC are totally independent of the study and should include a statistician	• the role of the DSMC is to assess the overall progress of the trial, and to monitor safety and critical efficacy endpoints • the DSMC should meet periodically during the trial and make recommendations to the Steering Committee on whether to continue, modify or stop a trial
Clinical Events Committee	• if appropriate, a Clinical Events Committee is appointed to adjudicate on clinical events • each pre-specified outcome is reviewed by an independent panel to ensure that they meet the definitions given in the trial protocol

TABLE 1. Trial organization in a multicenter trial

Ethical approval

All studies must be submitted to your Institutional Review Board or Independent Ethics Committee (IRB/IEC). You should determine how frequently your IRB/IEC meets. You will almost certainly need to submit the following documents:

- a finalized, signed original protocol with any protocol amendments
- any documents requiring patient involvement (e.g. patient diaries or questionnaires)
- an investigator's brochure and any safety information
- the investigator's curriculum vitae (CV)
- the patient information sheet tailored to local requirements
- the patient consent form
- any literature used for recruitment (e.g. advertisements)
- the investigator payment schedule
- information on patient payment or compensation
- regulatory documents pertaining to the investigational product (where applicable)

Indemnity and financial agreements

Prior to initiation of the trial at your center you must obtain insurance or indemnity agreements that provide insurance to indemnify the investigator (i.e. to secure against liability) and to compensate the patient in the event of a trial-related injury. The details of the indemnity agreement will vary from study to study. A signed agreement between the investigator and the sponsor (this may include details of the financial agreement) is also essential. The research services department and financial managers at your institution will need to approve this.

Study organization

It is important to liaise with colleagues as early as possible to discuss the study protocol and procedures on a one-to-one basis or in group training sessions, whichever is most appropriate.

It must be established who will screen, consent and randomize patients; an authorized person should always be available for these procedures. The sponsor will advise on whether the investigator alone may obtain consent from patients, or whether alternative personnel delegated by the investigator may do this in the investigator's absence. This is particularly important in studies involving acute admissions.

An area should be designated where the patient will be seen at your institution. For follow-up visits, establish who will see patients and perform study-related tests, procedures or measurements.

Specific tasks should be designated to appropriate individuals: e.g. responsibility for samples, scans or tests sent to a central laboratory (where applicable), or completion of the case report forms (CRFs) and study documentation (see chapter 7).

You may find a flow chart helpful to show which tests are required at each visit and any timelines for visit dates.

Systematic organization of a clinical trial is essential

It is important to:

1. liaise with colleagues as early as possible
2. identify the appropriate personnel for each task
3. establish appropriate locations for each task at your center

---

Training visits

Prior to commencement of the study, a training or initiation visit will take place at your site. You should ensure that all personnel involved in the study can attend and that all key study documentation is available for review (see below).

Following the training visit you should ensure that you are fully conversant with all study procedures including:

- eligibility criteria
- recruitment
- randomization
- dispensing of study drug or use of study device
- how to perform unblinding (if applicable)
- completion of the CRF and adverse event forms
- study measurements
- transport of samples

It is also essential to have a thorough understanding of the International Conference on Harmonisation Good Clinical Practice (ICH GCP) guideline.

Study documentation

In all studies a number of key documents must be completed and retained by the center and/or sponsor. These include:

- a finalized, signed original protocol (including the Declaration of Helsinki) and any amendments
- IRB/IEC approval letter and correspondence
- a copy of regulatory approval
  (the sponsor will provide this if applicable)
- a letter of indemnity (for insurance purposes)

- signed agreements between all parties (including financial agreements)
- CVs for the investigator, study team, laboratory director and pharmacist
- an authorized signatory list
- an investigator brochure
- a specimen patient consent form
- a specimen patient information sheet and any information given to the patient
- an advertisement for patient recruitment (if applicable)
- a specimen CRF
- a list of laboratory normal ranges, methods and accreditation/calibration certificates
- a trial training/initiation visit report
- instructions for use of the study drug or device (if not in the protocol)
- a method for emergency unblinding
- shipping records for the investigational product and certificate of analysis (where applicable)

Study awareness

The start-up phase should be used to increase awareness of the study. This can be done, e.g., by putting up posters summarizing the study, holding lunchtime seminars to give information to clinical colleagues, talking to patient support groups and submitting articles to patient support magazines (please note that you should ensure that you have obtained IRB/IEC consent prior to submission of any articles). Also, awareness can be increased by ensuring that colleagues are familiar with eligibility criteria.

It is recommended that you continue to raise awareness throughout the course of the study.

Screening and enrolment
Where do I find the patients I am looking for?

This will depend on the nature of the trial and the clinical question being asked. Guidance on screening and enrolment of patients is often provided in the protocol or other study documents. When deciding where to look for patients you should consider;

• the severity of their disease

Will your patients be found in general practitioners' surgeries or will they be hospital in-patients or out-patients?

• whether their disease is acute or chronic?

Patients with acute disease are likely to be admitted as hospital in-patients

• whether there is a specific location where you may find this patient population?

For example, renal patients in a dialysis unit, or post-myocardial infarction patients in a rehabilitation class

What is a screening log?

In some studies you will be asked to complete a log of all the potential patients screened for your trial. This should give details of whether or not the patients were enrolled in the study, and reasons for any exclusions. The screening log enables you and the coordinating center to monitor progression of the study and may help if you are finding it difficult to recruit patients (the log will show the reasons why and you will be able to discuss this with the sponsor). You may be asked to send this log to the sponsor at regular intervals.

How do I know if a patient is suitable for my study?

This depends on the eligibility criteria for the study. An examination of a patient's medical notes is advisable before approaching the patient. It is also a good idea to look up the results of any tests which could exclude the patient, and then to carry out any required tests (e.g. blood tests or X-rays).

You should have the patient's consent for any study-related investigations that are not a part of routine care.

Discuss the study with the patient. He/she may give you other reasons that render him/her unsuitable, such as participation in another study, an inability to comply with the study follow-up or personal reasons (e.g. their family situation prevents them taking part or the distance to travel is too great).

How should I approach a patient to gain informed consent?

There are a number of points to note when obtaining consent from patients:

- make sure that you are in a quiet place where you will not be disturbed
- describe the study clearly, detailing any potential benefits and side effects. Give the patient the patient information sheet
- go through the routine clinical practice for their condition and how your study may differ from this (e.g. any extra tests required)
- explain that they do not have to take part if they do not want to and that they are free to withdraw from the study at any point without giving a reason. This will not affect their subsequent medical care
- give the patient the opportunity to ask questions
- where possible you should give them time to think about participating, and to discuss the study with family and friends

- you will often be required to give the patient the contact details of an independent adviser who they can talk to about the study
- remember that consent forms should be signed in the presence of an authorized member of your study team. You must use a consent form that has been approved by the IRB/IEC. Many studies dictate that only doctors are authorized to obtain consent from patients, although study nurses and research coordinators may discuss the study with patients. The patient should retain a signed copy of the consent form

After the patient has given their consent and been enrolled into the study you should show them how to use the investigational product (if necessary) and give out any study materials (e.g. diaries). The patient should also be given a Study Identification Card detailing the study and a contact name and telephone number to use in case of any queries or problems. Follow-up visits can be arranged at this time if appropriate.

Meeting recruitment targets

When you agree to take part in a study you will agree to meet certain recruitment targets. If your actual recruitment rate is below your target rate then there are a number of ways to overcome this e.g. increasing your screening area and ensuring that all your colleagues are aware of the study. It may also be worth looking at how you have presented the study to patients; you may be confusing them. Sometimes it is useful to try a 'dummy run' of the consent procedure with a colleague.

Use of the investigational product

If a study involves a drug or device you will be required to complete an accountability form. This form will be study-specific. However, all accountability forms require a patient identifier (e.g. initials, date of birth or CRF number), date of dispensing/allocation and a product identifier (e.g. serial, lot or batch number) for each patient randomized. Also, if the study involves repeat visits you will need to record the date the product was returned and the amount of product taken (if a drug study) at each visit.

The accountability form should be signed at each visit by an authorized member of the study team and will be

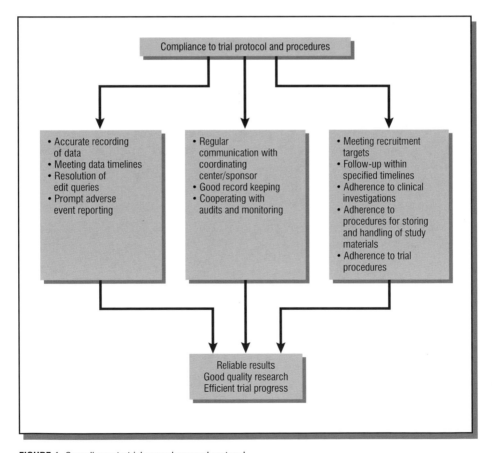

FIGURE 1. Compliance to trial procedures and protocol

checked by a study monitor from the coordinating center at subsequent visits.

You will be given instructions about the storage of drugs and devices (e.g. location in the institution, security and optimum temperature and humidity levels). It is your responsibility to ensure that they are stored in a safe place. In addition, any unblinding codes should be stored in a secure place that remains accessible to all members of the study team.

Compliance to trial procedures and protocol

It is vital that all procedures and activities described in the protocol are adhered to throughout the course of the study. Adhering to the protocol ensures reliable results, good quality research and efficient trial progress.

Follow-up

It is the responsibility of the participating center to ensure that patients are followed up in accordance with the protocol. All follow-up visits should be scheduled within the specified timelines. The patients must be made aware of procedures to be performed and the time these will take. It is also important to communicate with any departments assisting with follow-up, and to prepare a plan of action for any patients withdrawn from the study or who do not attend for follow-up.

It is possible that some patients will miss appointments, experience a change of circumstances or change contact details and become 'lost' in the follow-up phase. If patients do not attend for scheduled visits a number of strategies can be put in place to complete patient data collection, e.g.:

- contacting the patient by telephone
- organizing alternative attendance at local hospitals or GP practices

- arranging to send out questionnaires/diaries or other study materials if relevant
- contacting another family member if their details have been recorded
- obtaining information from the patient's hospital notes
- contacting GPs for data on adverse events

Attempts should be made to see these patients at least once after their withdrawal, to ensure safety of the patient and to recover any trial medications.

Identification and reporting of adverse events

An adverse event (AE) is defined as any untoward medical occurrence in a subject which does not necessarily have a causal relationship with the treatment. An AE may be classified as mild, moderate or severe.

Serious adverse events

A serious adverse event (SAE) is an AE which:

- results in death
- is life-threatening

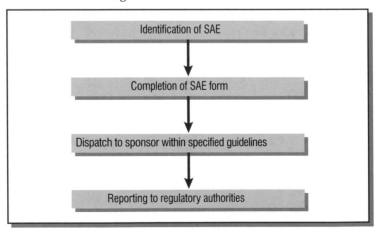

FIGURE 2. Reporting a SAE

- requires in-patient hospitalization (or prolongs existing hospitalization)
- results in persistent or significant disability or incapacity
- is a congenital anomaly or birth defect

The protocol will specify any additional trial-specific SAEs.

A **severe** AE is not the same as a **serious adverse event**.

The prompt and accurate reporting of any SAE is a protocol requirement in most studies and is essential for the safety of the trial participants. Specific forms will be provided for reporting SAEs.

Monitoring visits

The purpose of monitoring is to verify that the rights and well-being of patients are protected. This is done by ensuring that patients are recruited according to the protocol, that the consent procedure has been carried out correctly and that the patients fulfill all eligibility criteria.

In addition, all CRFs are checked during the monitoring visit for legibility, accuracy and completion of all data points. Some of these are then subjected to source data verification (SDV), which involves cross-checking the CRF against source data such as patient notes, diaries, questionnaires and test results to ensure accuracy and completeness of reporting.

How to prepare for a monitoring visit

When preparing for a monitoring visit you should:

- check that all the administrative paperwork is in order
- assemble all the source data required (e.g. patient notes and laboratory results)
- ensure that CRFs are clean and edit queries are resolved
- notify the pharmacy and relevant laboratories of the visit as the monitor may need to check these areas

- allow time for the study monitor to discuss any questions raised

Monitoring visits will also allow you to discuss any queries that have arisen that are not covered by the protocol.

Close-out activities

At trial termination a number of activities must be carried out including return of all completed CRFs (these may also be archived at the study site), unused CRFs, used or unused investigational products, code-breaking envelopes, equipment supplied and any outstanding documentation.

The investigator file must be complete. It is also your responsibility to ensure that data are archived in accordance with the sponsor's requirements.

Early termination of the trial

Early termination of a trial may occur as a result of, e.g., poor recruitment, inaccurate data collection, failure to meet data timelines or protocol violations. This action is a costly exercise and is always a last resort. However, centers will be closed if necessary to ensure data integrity and progress of the trial.

Remember by signing the agreement to participate in the trial, you undertake to carry out all activities as specified in the trial protocol.

Dos and don'ts of trial participation

Do

collect data accurately

respond quickly to quality control notes

report AEs and SAEs within agreed timelines

follow patients by scheduling return visits as required

have contingency plans for patients unable
to return to the center

keep the investigator file up to date

ask the coordinating center for advice if needed
on any trial procedure

Don't

think someone else will do it!

think errors will be missed by a trial monitor
or data manager

forget that the patient is the most important
aspect of the trial

Conclusion

Participation in a clinical trial, whether it be a single-center or multicenter trial, should be a beneficial experience. Clinical trials are an important way of providing information for evidence-based medicine. Involvement in a trial increases knowledge of the disease process under investigation and generally improves clinical practice standards and organization in participating hospitals. Furthermore, investigator meetings provide an opportunity to meet other health professionals and scientists with an interest in research. This allows the exchange of ideas and fosters future collaborations with the aim of improving health care.

CHAPTER 7
Case report forms and data management

Stephen Aldis & Fiona Nugara

Introduction

Data collected during a trial should be tailored to answer the hypothesis that is proposed within the protocol. To ensure that the 'correct data' are collected, a special form is designed called a case report form (also known as a case record form or CRF). Patient data from source documents such as the patient's medical records are used to complete CRFs. The completed forms are usually sent to a coordinating center responsible for the collection of trial data. The coordinating center will then ensure that the final data set is complete, accurate and complies with the study design.

What is a CRF?

The International Conference on Harmonisation Good Clinical Practice: Consolidated Guideline defines a CRF as:

"A *printed, optical or electronic document designed to record all of the protocol required information to be reported to the sponsor on each trial subject.*"

The completed CRF ensures that a standardized data set is collected for each trial subject.

Methods of data collection

The principal tool for data collection is the paper CRF; however, with the continual expansion of technology, data can now be collected in an electronic format as well. Electronic data capture methods will be covered later in this chapter.

What makes a good CRF?

The CRF is an essential tool for a clinical trial. A CRF designer will incorporate the views of medical staff, data managers/data entry staff, monitors, statisticians and investigators/study coordinators to ensure that the form is both easy to complete and collects all the necessary data.

What type of data will be collected?

The protocol broadly identifies the data that must be collected in order to achieve the study objectives and to meet regulatory requirements. Such data will include the following items:

- patient identification
- patient demographic details (e.g. age, sex, height)
- adherence to protocol inclusion/exclusion criteria
- baseline medical history
- diagnosis, indication for which the product is administered
- medications prior to procedure
- treatment details
- tracking of adverse and other key events
- discharge details
- follow-up visits

Format of a CRF

To ensure that the data requested in the CRF are collected accurately, the questions must be unambiguous and precise. Thus, the design should ensure that:

- *unnecessary data are not collected*

e.g., the collection of both date of birth and age

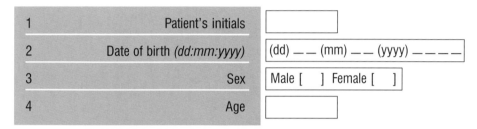

Duplication of data could lead to inconsistencies within the data and, therefore, create more work for both the study coordinator/investigator completing the forms and the data entry staff.

- *questions should be clear and concise*

- *definitions should be clear and easily understood*

7 ❤④ Documented myocardial infarction?	(dd) _ _ (mm) _ _ (yyyy) _ _ _ _

Documented acute myocardial infarction:
Two of the following three criteria must have been present:

1. unequivocal ECG changes
2. elevation of cardiac enzyme(s) above twice the upper limit of normal

8	History of diabetes mellitus (select only one)	Insulin dependent diabetes mellitus [ ] NIDDM – Treated with drugs [ ] NIDDM – Treated with diet [ ] No history of diabetes mellitus [ ]

3. chest pain typical of acute myocardial infarction which lasted more than 30 minutes

- *multiple choice format, free text must be avoided*
- *related data items are collated onto distinct CRF pages (e.g. baseline, treatment and follow-up phases)*

Serious adverse event forms

These special forms are designed to capture structured data on any serious side effects (see Chapter 6) of protocol treatment. Provision of these forms allows timely and accurate reporting of events.

Guidelines for completion of CRFs

The completion of CRFs will vary from trial to trial. However, there are some guidelines that are common to all trials. According to the ICH GCP guideline, CRFs must:

- be completed accurately and legibly, and reported in a timely manner
- correctly reflect the data found in the source documents
- have all questions answered, in an attempt to prevent the generation of data queries
- have any changes or corrections dated and initialed. These should not obscure the original entry, e.g.

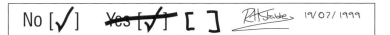

- be completed in accordance with the instructions for the trial, e.g.

No [ ] Yes [ ]	Answer by putting a tick mark in the appropriate box and proceed to the next line unless otherwise directed
No [*stop*] Yes [ ]	Putting a tick mark [4] in a box containing the word 'stop' means that you have encountered a protocol violation. Consult with the local investigators or the trial coordinating center
❤	If a ❤ follows a question this refers the investigator to specific instructions
Text	Must be entered in printed CAPITALS
Dates	Must be entered in day-month-year format, e.g. 19/07/1999

Details of all reported adverse events are sent to members of the independent Clinical Events Committee for adjudication to ensure that they meet study definitions. The results of the adjudication process are then entered onto the database. Once updated and validated, the database can be declared 'clean' and the data are subsequently analyzed by a statistician. The final report is then written.

Data Protection Act

The UK Data Protection Act became law on the 1st of March 2000, and at present it is unclear whether an exemption will be made for clinical trials. The impact of the act will include a requirement to incorporate information on data protection in the informed consent documentation. The patient may also have the right to review CRF data.

Electronic data capture

Many data management processes involve the use of clinical trial database systems that 'capture' data electronically. The important features of electronic data capture (EDC) systems are:

• electronic case report forms (eCRF)

Data entry screens that provide a graphical user interface (GUI) to enter data into the trial database (these screens should look as similar as possible to the paper CRF pages to facilitate easier data entry)

• consistency checks (within a form and between forms)

Logical checks and rules that increase data validity and consistency, e.g. if a systolic blood pressure entry falls outside a pre-determined range, an automatic request will be made to confirm the entry

• schedule information

The chronological ordering of CRF pages and the timeframe in which they are due

• security – user/task permissions (who's permitted to do what)

For example, a research nurse entering data at one particular trial site should have permission to view data from that site only and no others

• full audit capabilities

Every data item value that is entered as part of the trial should have a date and time stamp, and a user identification associated with it. This provides an audit trail for tracking any changes and the personnel involved in making those changes.

• reporting

To achieve a 'clean' data set, the inconsistencies and missing CRF pages generated through the checking facilities must be reported to the trial site.

Many of the features of EDC are implemented to ensure that the system is FDA and ICH GCP compliant.

Paper versus electronic data capture
Paper CRFs

Advantages

• With two part No Carbon Required (NCR) CRFs,
  a second copy of the data will be recorded. Copies of
  the data can be retained at the study site as well as
  at the coordinating center
• Universal access

Disadvantages

- Completed CRFs must be archived in accordance with regulatory requirements
- The data recorded on CRFs require subsequent central data entry
- There is potential for error when the data entry staff transcribe the data from the paper CRFs to the trial database

Electronic data capture

Advantages

- Time-consuming phases of the trial can be automated (e.g. data validation and data query reporting)
- Audit trails (records changes made to the data throughout the study)
- Remote data entry ensures 'real time' data acquisition from center

Disadvantages

- Development of stand-alone software may be very expensive
- Operators of EDC systems require extensive training
- Requires technology in place at study sites
- Providing full compliance with industry and regulatory standards can be expensive

Method	Description
Local client/server[1]	Paper CRFs sent to the data coordinating center are entered through a GUI (client) into the central database. Logical inconsistency checks are 'run' against the data and any inconsistencies are raised and reported to the trial site
Remote data entry (RDE)	Remote data entry is a method by which the data are captured (entered) at source, e.g. the hospital clinic. Logical inconsistencies are thus raised also at source, thereby ensuring that the data can be reviewed at a much earlier stage. RDE exists in two models:
	• **Off-line (distributed client/server[1])** – similar to the local client/server model. Data are entered into a copy of the central database at the local trial site. Periodically the local trial site 'uploads' the data, usually via a modem, and synchronizes the data at the coordinating center
	• **On-line (internet-based)** – data are entered directly into eCRFs that are web pages. Consistency checks are executed against the data that are entered and the completed eCRF updates the central database. Internet RDE is the only true 'real time' RDE electronic data capture method
Data capture from optical images	Paper CRF pages sent to the central coordinating center are scanned to provide a digital image. Depending on the format of the CRF pages, one or more of the following recognition techniques is applied to the optical image. The information elucidated from the optical image provides the data for the CRF page.
	• Optical mark recognition (OMR) – OMR decodes marks on the optical image, e.g. a cross entered into a check box on a CRF page
	• Optical character recognition (OCR) – OCR decodes characters and numbers on the optical image. Usually, the characters and numbers are in a defined area of the form
	• Intelligent character recognition (ICR) – ICR is used in conjunction with OCR. If a character cannot be matched, an 'intelligent' guess is made from data acquired from previous recognition sessions (the algorithms utilized in ICR are very complex)
	• Unfortunately, the accuracy of the three recognition processes detailed above rarely achieves 100%, therefore it is still necessary to enter and check data values manually
Fax-based data capture	This form of EDC is a heterogeneous combination of the methods described previously. The paper CRFs are faxed from the trial site and subsequently the CRF is either printed out and entered manually through a GUI, or the fax provides the optical image for one of the recognition processes described previously.

[1] Applications running on a (client) computer may access data stored on another (server) computer.
CRF: case report form; eCRF: electronic case report form; EDC: electronic data capture; GUI: graphical user interface; ICR: intelligent character recognition; OCR: optical character recognition; OMR: optical mark recognition; RDE: remote data entry

TABLE 1. Methods of electronic data capture

Conclusion

This chapter provides an overview of the systems that must be implemented and the resources required to provide quality data and concise reporting. Good design and planning are critical to the success of a clinical trial. The design of CRFs, whether on paper or in an electronic format, will help to ensure the collection of good quality, reliable data. Data generated in a trial have to undergo extensive checking to ensure completeness, consistency and accuracy. Ensuring data quality is a process best managed by an experienced coordinating center. However, the most reliable information in clinical trials comes from committed well-trained investigators and study coordinators at participating sites who provide, within agreed timelines, the data necessary for a successful trial.

▌INDEX

K

Kaplan-Meier analysis, defined 37–38

L

laboratories
    clinical trial responsibilities of staff 56–57
    cost considerations 58, 61
learning curve effect, interventional procedures 17
Local Research Ethics Committee (LREC) 50

M

marketing authorization (MA)
    applications 43
    commitments post-authorization 44
Medwatch
    USA, post-MA authorization commitments 44
    web site 52
monitoring visits 75–76
Multi-Centre Research Ethics Committee (MREC), web site 48, 52
multicenter trials
    design issues 63–77
    documentation 67–68
    enrolment and screening 69
    ethical approval 65
    indemnity agreements and financial considerations 65
    participation 63–77
        close-out activities 76
        organization 64, 66
        study awareness 68
    recruitment targets 71
multivariate/univariate analysis, defined 35

N

New Drug Application (NDA), MA application, USA 43
normal distribution see statistical normality
number needed to treat (NNT), defined 36

O

objective defined studies 40–41
observational studies, design issues 1–14
odds ratio (OR), defined 35–36